STOIC STRENGTH

The Philosophy of Fitness and Resilience

Matheus Lourenco

CONTENTS

INTRODUCTION: A JOURNEY TO RESILIENCE

"The impediment to action advances action. What stands in the way becomes the way." — **Marcus Aurelius**

Welcome to *Stoic Strength: The Philosophy of Fitness and Resilience*. This isn't just another fitness book. It's an invitation to transform not only your body but your mindset—an opportunity to align your physical efforts with the timeless wisdom of Stoicism.

Stoicism has endured for centuries because its lessons are universal. At its core are four guiding virtues:

- **Wisdom:** Making informed, thoughtful decisions about your health and fitness, focusing on what truly matters.
- **Courage:** Facing discomfort, pushing through challenges, and finding strength in moments of doubt.
- **Justice:** Honoring your commitments to yourself and others while living with fairness and integrity.
- **Temperance:** Striking a balance in all you do, avoiding extremes, and cultivating sustainable habits.

When we bring these principles into our fitness journey,

something incredible happens. Training becomes more than a physical activity. It becomes a practice in resilience, self-discipline, and mental clarity. Every rep, every challenge, every setback becomes a tool for growth.

Why This Book?

Whether you're an experienced athlete, returning to fitness after a break, or stepping into this world for the first time, you've likely faced obstacles. Maybe it's a lack of motivation. Maybe it's fear of failure. Or maybe life just keeps getting in the way.

This book is here to remind you: those obstacles aren't barriers to your progress—they're steppingstones, The same challenges that frustrate you today are the ones that will build your strength tomorrow.

What You'll Learn

Throughout these pages, we'll explore how Stoic philosophy can help you:

- Cultivate discipline and consistency, even on the toughest days.
- Embrace adversity and use it as fuel for growth.
- Balance ambition with patience, avoiding burnout.
- Strengthen not just your body, but your mind and spirit.

Each chapter blends practical fitness strategies with Stoic teachings, showing you how to navigate setbacks, build habits that last, and grow stronger in every sense of the word.

CHAPTER 1: STOIC FOUNDATIONS FOR FITNESS

"You have power over your mind—not outside events. Realize this, and you will find strength." — **Marcus Aurelius**

Every fitness journey starts the same way: with a decision. A moment when you choose to become something more. You might not feel ready. You might not know where to start. But what matters isn't what you lack—it's the choice you make to begin. That's where strength is born.

For centuries, the Stoics have offered wisdom for navigating life's challenges with clarity, resilience, and purpose. At its core, fitness is no different. The gym, the track, the weights—they aren't just tools for physical growth. They are arenas where you test your character, sharpen your discipline, and build a version of yourself capable of more than you imagined.

This book isn't about quick fixes or shortcuts. It's not about perfection. It's about a way of life. One that draws from timeless principles to guide you through every obstacle and every triumph.

Why Stoicism? Why Fitness?

At first glance, ancient philosophy and modern fitness might seem worlds apart. But the Stoics understood something we often forget: the pursuit of strength begins in the mind. Fitness isn't just a physical act; it's a mental one. When you lift a weight, you're not just training your body—you're training your will. When you push through discomfort, you're building resilience. When you choose consistency over excuses, you're proving to yourself what's possible.

Fitness and Stoicism are both about action. About showing up, doing the work, and accepting the challenges as part of the process. This philosophy is not something you simply think about —it's something you practice.

The Journey Ahead

This book is your guide. Through it, you will discover how the Stoic virtues of Wisdom, Courage, Justice, and Temperance can transform not just your workouts, but your mindset, your habits, and your life.

Wisdom
Epictetus wrote, "A fool is known by his speech; and a wise man by his silence." Wisdom will help you focus on what truly matters and let go of what doesn't.

Courage
Marcus Aurelius wrote, "It is not death that a man should fear, but he should fear never beginning to live." Courage will teach you to face discomfort, fear, and failure with strength.

Justice

Seneca wrote, "The willing are led by fate, the reluctant are dragged." Justice will remind you to honor your commitments and hold yourself accountable.

Temperance

Zeno of Citium wrote, "Better to trip with the feet than with the tongue." Temperance will guide you to balance effort and rest, intensity and sustainability.

Each chapter will offer tools to overcome obstacles, reframe challenges, and build the discipline you need to succeed. There are no secrets here—just principles that work when you commit to them.

Begin Where You Are

You don't need the perfect plan. You don't need the perfect moment. You just need to begin. The weight you lift today, the steps you take today, are enough. Progress is not measured by perfection, but by movement.

Ask yourself: Why am I doing this? Hold on to that answer. Because when the days get hard—and they will—that reason will keep you moving forward.

This isn't just about fitness. It's about building the kind of strength that carries you through life. The obstacles ahead are not there to stop you—they are there to shape you.

Welcome to the journey. Let's begin.

"Strength is not born in grand gestures, but in the quiet

decision to begin." — Matheus Lourenco

From Mindset to Movement

A stoic mindset lays the foundation, but it's discipline that builds the structure. Let's dive into how to turn intention into action.

CHAPTER 2: DISCIPLINE IN ACTION

Do every act of your life as though it were the very last act of your life" — **Marcus Aurelius**

Discipline and action are two sides of the same coin. Discipline gives us the framework to succeed, while action breathes life into our intentions. Yet, the greatest obstacle between intention and execution is often procrastination. The Stoics understood this dynamic deeply, teaching that progress requires both the steadiness of discipline and the courage to act.

The Foundation: Discipline As A Habit

Discipline is not a burst of motivation; it's the steady commitment to show up, regardless of how you feel. Marcus Aurelius reminds us, "You have power over your mind—not outside events. Realize this, and you will find strength." The mind is where discipline begins, and building it is a process of repeated effort.

Practical Step: Identify one habit that aligns with your goals and focus on mastering it daily. Whether it's committing to a specific workout or setting aside time to write, consistency creates momentum.

Overcoming Emotional Barriers

Procrastination often stems from fear: fear of failure, imperfection, or even success. Epictetus said, "Men are disturbed not by things, but by the views they take of them." By addressing the emotions behind procrastination, we reclaim our ability to act.

Practical Step: When faced with procrastination, pause and identify the underlying emotion. Write it down and reframe it: instead of viewing the task as overwhelming, see it as an opportunity to grow.

Break Tasks Into Small Steps

Large goals can feel daunting, creating a sense of paralysis. The Stoics teach us to focus on the present moment and the action within our control. Marcus Aurelius advises, "Do what is necessary. Then do what is possible.

Practical Step: Take the first step, however small. If writing a report feels overwhelming, start with a single sentence. If a workout seems impossible, begin with a stretch or a warm-up. Action defeats inertia.

Detach From Perfection

Perfectionism is a hidden form of procrastination. The fear that our efforts won't measure up keeps us stagnant. Seneca reminds us, "It is not because things are difficult that we do not dare; it is because we do not dare that they are difficult."

Practical Step: Focus on progress, not perfection. Allow yourself to make mistakes, knowing that effort builds mastery over time.

The Interplay Of Discipline And Action

Discipline provides the framework, but action is what turns potential into reality. Together, they create a cycle of progress: discipline builds the habit of showing up, and action reinforces the value of effort.

Practical Step: Combine structure with flexibility. Plan your day with clear blocks of time for focused action, but remain adaptable when challenges arise. Treat each completed task as a small victory.

Real Life Example: Turning Procrastination Into Progress

There was a time when I kept putting off starting a structured workout plan. I'd always tell myself, "I'll start on Monday," but when Monday came, there was always an excuse—a busy day at work, feeling tired, or even convincing myself that I'd just start the next week instead.

One day, I realized something: waiting for the "perfect time" was just a way of staying comfortable. So, I made a deal with myself: no more overthinking, no more excuses—just 10 minutes of movement. If I felt like stopping after 10 minutes, I could, but I had to start.

That small decision changed everything. I showed up, pushed through those first 10 minutes, and usually ended up completing the entire session. The momentum from that one choice—to act instead of waiting—created a habit that stuck.

The lesson? Discipline isn't about being perfect or waiting for the ideal moment. It's about taking the smallest action, no matter how you feel. Once you start, the rest becomes easier.

Reflection

Ask yourself: What emotions or thoughts have been holding me back from taking action? How can I begin now, without waiting for the perfect moment?

Remember, the greatest obstacle to action often lies within. By confronting our inner barriers with courage and clarity, we take the first step toward transforming intentions into reality. Every small action is an act of defiance against procrastination and a step toward growth.

"Success begins when you stop asking how you feel and start focusing on what needs to be done." — Matheus Lourenco

From Action to Self-Control

Discipline turns ideas into actions, but self-control sustains them. In the next chapter, we'll explore how mastering impulses can lead to greater freedom and long-term success.

CHAPTER 3: SELF-CONTROL IN MOTION

"No man is free who is not master of himself." — **Epictetus**

Self-control is the cornerstone of success in both Stoicism and fitness. It is the ability to govern your impulses, align your actions with your values, and make decisions that prioritize long-term goals over fleeting desires. In fitness, self-control is what keeps you showing up for workouts when motivation wanes, choosing nutritious meals over indulgent ones, and staying disciplined in the face of challenges. It's not just about restraint—it's about mastery.

Cultivating Self-Control In Fitness

Set Clear and Meaningful Goals
Epictetus reminds us that freedom comes from self-mastery, and self-control becomes far easier when guided by a purpose. Define what success looks like for you. Is it better health? Greater strength? Confidence in your abilities? These goals act as your compass, keeping you grounded and motivated when the path gets difficult.

Embrace Delayed Gratification

The results you seek in fitness—whether it's a stronger body, increased stamina, or improved mental clarity—aren't immediate. And that's okay. The ability to delay gratification is a hallmark of self-control. Skip the sugary dessert today for the energy and vitality you'll feel tomorrow. Push through the final reps of a workout because you know they bring you closer to your vision. Every moment of discipline is an investment in your future self.

Build Habits That Reinforce Self-Control

Habits are self-control on autopilot. The more you can systematize your routines, the less you'll need to rely on sheer willpower. Schedule your workouts at the same time each day. Prep your meals in advance. Over time, these habits become second nature, making it easier to stay consistent even on tough days.

A Stoic Test Of Temptation

Imagine you're at a celebration surrounded by tempting foods and drinks. Everyone around you is indulging, and you feel the pull to do the same. Here's the Stoic approach: pause, reflect, and align your choices with your goals. Maybe you enjoy a small treat to partake in the moment but avoid excess that derails your progress. Balance isn't weakness; it's wisdom. Self-control doesn't mean abstaining from joy—it means enjoying life on your own terms.

"Freedom is the only worthy goal in life. It is won by disregarding things that lie beyond our control." — **Epictetus**

Real Life Example: Mastering Your Reactions

A few years ago, I heard someone laughing and making fun of my form. For a quick moment, I felt a rush of anger. I wanted to turn around, say something, or prove them wrong. But instead, I stopped, took a deep breath, and focused on why I was there.

The gym wasn't about them—it was about me. I tuned out their voices, finished my set, and kept going. By the end of the session, their words didn't matter anymore. What mattered was that I didn't let them control me.

That moment stayed with me. It reminded me that self-control isn't about ignoring how you feel—it's about choosing how to act. Every time you decide to stay calm, you're building a strength that goes far beyond the gym.

Reflection: Mastering Self-Control

Take a moment to examine your fitness journey with clarity. Where do your impulses challenge your progress the most? Is it skipping workouts when you're tired? Giving in to indulgent meals when stress hits? Use the Stoic principle of reflection as a tool for action: pause, observe, and ask yourself—what patterns are holding me back?

Self-control begins with awareness. Epictetus reminds us that while we can't always control external triggers, we can control how we respond. By identifying the root causes of your struggles, you gain the power to choose better actions, one decision at a time.

"If you are distressed by anything external, the pain is not due to the thing itself but to your estimate of it; and this you have the power to revoke at any moment." — Marcus Aurelius

Embrace Discomfort, Embrace Growth

Discomfort is not the enemy—it's the price of progress. Stoicism teaches us to reframe discomfort as an opportunity to grow. In fitness, this means leaning into challenges. Lift heavier weights. Run farther. Stretch longer. Push beyond what feels easy. Growth lies on the other side of discomfort, and self-control is what helps you get there.

By mastering self-control, you unlock the true freedom to live according to your values and achieve your goals. In fitness, as in life, the battle is within—and victory is always within reach.

"True power is not found in what you can conquer, but in how well you can govern yourself." — Matheus Lourenco

From Self-Control to Flexibility

Self-control strengthens your resolve, but true growth demands adaptability. In the next chapter, we'll explore how mental and emotional flexibility can transform obstacles into opportunities.

CHAPTER 4: FLEXIBILITY IN MIND AND EMOTION

"Man conquers the world by conquering himself." — **Zeno of Citium**

Life rarely goes as planned. A project falls apart. A relationship changes. You set a goal, but something gets in the way. These moments can feel overwhelming, but they don't have to. The Stoics remind us that strength isn't about rigidity—it's about adaptability.

Flexibility isn't a sign of weakness; it's the foundation of resilience. It's what allows us to adjust, to bend without breaking, and to find a new way forward when things don't go as expected. When you learn to let go of what you can't control and embrace change, you stop fighting against life—and start working with it.

The Art Of Letting Go

One of the hardest lessons in life is knowing when to let go. We cling to old plans, failed goals, and even past versions of ourselves, hoping to regain what's already gone. But holding on doesn't help us move forward—it keeps us stuck.

Imagine you're training for a marathon, but halfway through, an injury forces you to stop running. It's frustrating. But instead of obsessing over what you can't do, you could shift your focus. Maybe this is a chance to build strength through weight training or improve flexibility with yoga. By letting go of what's no longer possible, you create space for new opportunities.

Letting go isn't about giving up—it's about adapting. It's recognizing when a path has reached its end and having the courage to take another.

Simple Strategies For Flexibility

The Stoics left us with practical tools to help navigate life's challenges. Here are three that can help you cultivate mental and emotional flexibility:

1. Shift Your Perspective

When faced with a challenge, step back and ask: *"How else can I see this?"* Maybe the setback isn't a failure—it's an opportunity to grow. A missed workout could be a chance to rest. A tough conversation might strengthen a relationship. Shifting your perspective helps you see solutions instead of obstacles.

2. Prepare for the Unexpected

The Stoics used the phrase *"if circumstances allow"* to remind themselves that life is unpredictable. Make your plans, but stay ready to adapt. If one door closes, look for another.

3. Reflect on What Truly Matters

Take a moment to think about what you value most. Are you holding onto something just because it feels safe? Letting go doesn't mean you lose—it means you make room for what's really important.

Why Flexibility Matters

Flexibility isn't just about fitness—it's about life. It's the skill that helps you navigate everything from missed goals to unexpected changes. It allows you to pivot without losing your sense of direction, to adjust without feeling defeated.

Think of it like water: it doesn't resist obstacles; it flows around them. Flexibility lets you do the same. It helps you move forward, no matter what stands in your way.

Real Life Example: Starting Over In A New City

When I moved to a new city, it felt like my entire world had shifted. My routine vanished—my gym, my running routes, my social life, and even the familiarity of how things used to work. Like I was starting from scratch.

I missed the comfort of my old life—the friends I could call without thinking twice and the gym that felt like a second home. But instead of letting frustration take over, I chose to focus on small steps forward.

So I joined a new gym, even though it felt awkward at first. I explored different running routes, getting lost more times than I'd like to admit. At work, I pushed myself to connect with colleagues and start building new friendships. Slowly, those small efforts started to add up.

That experience showed me that flexibility is more than changing your routine—it's about shifting your mindset. Life will always throw changes at you, but how you respond determines whether you stay stuck or keep moving forward.

Reflection

Ask yourself:

- *Am I holding onto something that's no longer serving me?*
- *How can I approach this challenge with more flexibility?*
- *What opportunities might open up if I let go?*

Flexibility isn't about being passive—it's about being adaptable. It's about trusting that no matter how life shifts, you can handle it.

"You can't control everything, but you can control how you respond. Stay flexible, and you'll always find a way forward."

Growth is not about avoiding change but about learning to flow with it." — Matheus Lourenco

From Flexibility to Patience

Flexibility teaches us to adapt to challenges, but patience allows us to endure the slow progress of growth. Let's explore how cultivating patience can transform your fitness journey and your mindset.

CHAPTER 5:
PERSISTENCE
AND PACIENCE

"Patience is the companion of wisdom." — **Seneca**

Patience As Strength

"No great thing is created suddenly, any more than a bunch of grapes or a fig. If you tell me that you desire a fig, I answer you that there must be time. Let it first blossom, then bear fruit, then ripen." — *Epictetus*

Progress is rarely immediate. It's easy to feel frustrated when results don't come as quickly as we hoped. But true growth—whether in fitness, life, or character—requires patience. The Stoics teach us that strength isn't just about endurance; it's about trusting the process and staying present, even when progress feels invisible.

Imagine planting a tree. You water it daily, ensure it gets sunlight, and protect it from harm. For weeks, maybe months, nothing seems to happen. But beneath the surface, roots are spreading, anchoring the tree, preparing it to grow. The same is true for your journey. The effort you put in today might not bear fruit immediately, but it's laying the foundation for results that will last.

Appreciate Progress Along The Way

Seneca reminds us: "He who is brave is free." In the context of persistence, bravery often looks like showing up, day after day, even when progress feels slow. And one of the most powerful tools to fuel that bravery is recognizing and celebrating small victories along the way.

Ran an extra mile? Lifted a heavier weight? Stayed consistent for a week? These moments might seem small, but they're proof of your progress. Each one is a step forward, a root growing deeper. Acknowledge them. They're the milestones that keep you moving forward.

Trust The Process

Marcus Aurelius wrote: "Look within. Within is the fountain of good, and it will ever bubble up if thou wilt ever dig." Persistence requires faith in the process. It means accepting that the results you want are a byproduct of consistent effort, not a reward for perfection.

The gym is a perfect teacher of this lesson. Some days you feel strong; other days, every lift feels heavy. But persistence is about showing up anyway. It's about recognizing that progress isn't linear but cumulative. Over time, the days you thought didn't matter will add up to something extraordinary.

Reframe Setbacks

Epictetus reminds us: "Difficulties show a person's character. Therefore, when a difficulty falls upon you, remember that God, like a trainer of wrestlers, has matched you with a rough young man."

Setbacks are not failures; they're lessons. Missed workouts, plateaus, or unexpected challenges are opportunities to adjust your approach and grow stronger. Instead of seeing them as proof that you're failing, view them as tests—chances to practice resilience and adapt.

Real-Life Example: Learning To Be Patient

When I first started strength training, I was eager to see results. I thought that after a few weeks, I'd notice big changes in my body. But as the days turned into weeks, and the weeks into months, the progress felt painfully slow. At one point, I started questioning if it was even worth it. I wanted to quit.

But instead of giving up, I reminded myself why I started. So I kept showing up at the gym, even on the days I didn't feel like it, and focused on the process instead of the results. Months later, I looked back and realized how far I had come—not just physically, but mentally. The small, consistent efforts I made each day had added up in ways I couldn't see in the moment. Patience isn't easy, but it's the key to real growth. The results you want will come— not overnight, but through persistence and trust in the process."

Reflection

Ask yourself:

Am I celebrating the small victories that prove my progress?

How can I reframe today's challenges as opportunities to grow?

Am I showing up for the process, even when progress feels slow?

Persistence is the art of trusting yourself—of believing that the roots you're planting today will one day support something extraordinary. The Stoics teach us that the journey is the reward, and every step along the way shapes who we are becoming.

"Patience and persistence are the two greatest warriors."

"Patience is the strength to trust the process, even when results seem distant." — Matheus Lourenco

From Patience to Reflection

Patience teaches us to trust the process, but reflection helps us refine it. In the next chapter, we'll explore how introspection can sharpen your fitness journey and align it with your core values.

CHAPTER 6: REFLECTION FOR GROWTH

"Let each thing you do, say, or intend be like that of a dying man." — Marcus Aurelius

Reflection is the mirror that reveals progress—or the lack of it. For the Stoics, reflection was not merely an occasional act but a daily practice, essential to self-improvement. In the realm of fitness, reflection helps refine your approach, align your actions with your goals, and uncover the gaps between intention and execution.

Reflection As A Tool For Growth

Seneca said, "We suffer more often in imagination than in reality." Reflection allows you to separate imagined barriers from real ones. By assessing your performance, you gain clarity about what works and what doesn't, whether in training, diet, or recovery.

Practical Step: After each workout, ask yourself: What went well? What could I improve? This habit will help you adjust your efforts and avoid repeating mistakes.

Aligning Fitness With Values

The Stoics believed in living a life consistent with one's values. In fitness, this means asking whether your actions reflect your deeper intentions. Are you training for health, for strength, or for vanity? The answer shapes your journey.

Practical Step: Write down your fitness goals and ask: Are these goals aligned with my values? If not, refine them until they resonate with your true purpose.

Daily Reflection For Mental Clarity

Epictetus taught, "Examine yourself, for it is your own responsibility." Reflection isn't just about the physical—it sharpens the mind. A daily practice of introspection keeps you grounded, focused, and resilient, both in the gym and in life.

Practical Step: At the end of each day, reflect on three questions:

What did I do well today?

What could I have done better?

What will I focus on tomorrow

Real Life Example: Learning From Setbacks

There was a time when I failed to hit a major fitness goal I had set for myself. I hit the gym hard, followed my routine, and pushed through difficult days, but when the deadline came, I fell short. In the first few days, I was frustrated and disappointed, questioning if all the effort was really worth it.

Instead of ignoring how I felt, I sat down to reflect. I asked myself tough questions: What went wrong? Did I overestimate what I could achieve? Was my approach realistic? Through that process, I realized I had been so focused on intensity that I'd neglected consistency. Some days, I pushed too hard and burned out, which set me back more than I realized.

From that reflection, I adjusted my goals, created a more sustainable plan, and focused on building habits that lasted. The next time I set a goal, I surpassed it—not because I worked harder, but because I worked smarter.

That experience showed me that setbacks aren't failures—they're opportunities to learn and grow. Reflection isn't about dwelling on mistakes—it's about turning them into stepping stones for progress.

Reflection

Ask yourself: Am I taking time to reflect on my journey? Do my actions align with my goals and values? Reflection is not an indulgence—it is a necessity. It keeps you honest, focused, and moving forward on the path of progress.

True growth requires not just effort, but the clarity to understand what's working and what's not." — Matheus Lourenco

From Reflection to Environment

Reflection gives us clarity about our inner world, but the environment we live in often shapes our external progress. Let's explore how your surroundings influence your growth and how you can intentionally craft an environment that supports your goals.

CHAPTER 7: ENVIRONMENT AND PROGRESS

"The soul becomes dyed with the color of its thoughts."— **Marcus Aurelius**

Your environment is not just a backdrop to your actions—it's the stage on which your progress is built. The Stoics knew that while you cannot always control your circumstances, you can shape what surrounds you to support your growth. Whether it's the people in your life, the spaces you inhabit, or the routines you follow, your environment whispers to you every day. The question is: what is it saying?

The Power Of Your Environment

Your environment silently shapes your habits, decisions, and progress. Take a closer look at your surroundings: Are they helping or hindering your growth? Reflect on the routines you follow, the spaces where you train, and the people you interact with daily.

Small adjustments can create a powerful impact. Rearrange your workspace for focus. Organize your kitchen to encourage healthy choices. Seek out people who inspire you to stay consistent. A well-designed environment does more than support your progress—it eliminates excuses.

The Influence Of Others

Seneca wrote, "Associate with those who will make a better man of you." The company you keep shapes your character more than you realize. Positive influences lift you higher, while negative ones weigh you down. Relationships, like environments, either build or erode your strength.

Reflection: Who do you spend your time with? Are they helping you move toward your goals, or pulling you away? Seek out those who challenge you to grow, and distance yourself from those who anchor you in the past.

Small Adjustments, Big Changes

The Stoics believed in intentionality. By making small changes to your environment, you can create significant shifts in your behavior. Epictetus taught, "Practice yourself, for heaven's sake, in little things, and then proceed to greater." A slight tweak—like setting up your workout clothes the night before or limiting access to social media during work hours—can be the difference between stagnation and progress.

Reflection: What small change can you make today to eliminate friction in your life? Progress often begins with the removal of obstacles.

The Inner Environment

While the external world shapes you, your inner environment is just as powerful. Epictetus reminds us, "We cannot choose our external circumstances, but we can always choose how we respond to them." A resilient mindset is built by cultivating gratitude, focus, and purpose in the face of any environment.

Music, too, can be a powerful tool for shaping your inner environment. The right playlist transforms a challenging workout into an act of purpose and focus, drowning out distractions and helping you connect with the rhythm of effort. Use music not just as background noise, but as an intentional element that enhances your mindset and elevates your performance.

Reflection: Begin each day with a simple question: What do I have today that supports my goals? Gratitude clears the mind and anchors you in the present.

Real Life Example: Outgrowing Old Circles

When I started changing my habits—waking up early to train, eating better, and focusing on my goals—I noticed something unexpected. Some of my closest friendships began to fade.

At first, I felt really guilty and i wondered if I was being selfish or something. But at some time I noticed it wasn't about me or them being better or worse than me but was just our paths that were no longer the same.

While I was prioritizing discipline and growth, they were still focused on nights out and familiar routines. And that's okay. Growing apart doesn't mean cutting people off—it simply means making space for the things that help you grow.

That lesson wasn't easy, but it was freeing. It taught me that not everyone is meant to stay in your life forever. Sometimes, growth means letting go—not with resentment, but with gratitude for the part they played in your story.

Reflection

Take a moment to assess the spaces, people, and routines that fill your life. Are they aligned with the person you want to become? Your environment whispers to you every day—make sure it's a voice that strengthens, not weakens, your resolve.

"Surround yourself with what inspires you, and let go of what no longer serves your journey." — Matheus Lourenco

From Environment to Mental Barriers

Your environment shapes your external progress, but the most challenging battles are fought within. In the next chapter, we'll explore how to overcome the mental barriers that hold you back and unlock your full potential.

CHAPTER 8: BREAKING MENTAL BARRIERS

"The greater the obstacle, the more glory in overcoming it." — **Molière**

Barriers, real or imagined, are inevitable in any fitness journey. Some are physical—like a plateau or an injury. But the most persistent obstacles are the ones we create in our own minds. These mental barriers whisper doubts, magnify failures, and convince us that progress is out of reach. The Stoics teach us that the path to strength, both physical and mental, is not about avoiding these barriers, but confronting and overcoming them.

Reframe The Challenge

Epictetus reminds us: "Men are disturbed not by things, but by the views they take of them." The way we perceive a challenge determines our ability to overcome it. When faced with a daunting workout, a lack of progress, or even the fear of failure, the first step is to shift perspective. Ask yourself: What can I learn from this? How can this make me stronger?

Reframing doesn't erase the difficulty, but it redefines its purpose. A hard workout becomes a test of character. A bad day becomes an opportunity to practice resilience. Each challenge is not a setback but a stepping stone, waiting for you to step up.

Train For The Worst, Expect The Best

Marcus Aurelius advises: "If you are distressed by anything external, the pain is not due to the thing itself but to your estimate of it; and this you have the power to revoke at any moment." Mental barriers often arise from fear of the unknown—what if I fail? What if I'm not good enough?

Instead of simply visualizing success, prepare for resistance. Anticipate discomfort, fatigue, or even failure, and decide how you will respond. If you're ready for the worst, you're less likely to be shaken when it comes. And when success arrives, it will be all the more rewarding because you've earned it.

Find Strength In Failure

Seneca said: "Every new beginning comes from some other beginning's end." Failure is not the enemy; it's the teacher. Each missed lift, skipped workout, or setback is a chance to adjust, refine, and grow stronger.

Real growth comes when you analyze failure without judgment. Instead of seeing it as evidence of your limits, view it as feedback. What went wrong? How can you improve? By embracing failure as part of the process, you turn every stumble into a step forward.

Real-Life Example: Changing The Story To Overcome Fear

There was a time when I avoided heavy deadlifts because of

a small incident years ago. I'd tried lifting more than I could handle back then, and the bar barely moved off the floor. It felt humiliating at the time, and I carried that memory with me every time I saw a loaded barbell.

One day, I realized this wasn't about the weight—it was about the story I'd been telling myself. I decided to stop avoiding it and face it head-on. I started light, focusing on form, adding just a little more weight each session. Every successful lift chipped away at that fear until one day, I hit a personal best I never thought possible.

That experience taught me a key lesson: mental barriers aren't about what you can or can't do—they're about what you believe. When you change the story, you change what's possible."*

Reflection

The greatest battles in fitness are fought in the mind. Barriers will come, but how you choose to approach them makes all the difference. Ask yourself:

Am I letting fear or doubt dictate my actions?
What mental barriers are holding me back from progress?
How can I reframe today's challenge as tomorrow's opportunity?

The Stoics remind us that obstacles are not meant to stop us. They are meant to shape us. Each barrier you face is a chance to grow stronger, more resilient, and more determined. Use these moments not as excuses to quit, but as reasons to persist.

"When you master your inner battles, the obstacles outside

lose their power." — Matheus Lourenco

From Mental Barriers to Emotional Mastery

Breaking through mental barriers helps us see our potential, but mastering emotions allows us to harness that potential fully. In the next chapter, we'll explore how emotional control can fuel both your fitness journey and your personal growth.

CHAPTER 9: EMOTIONAL MASTERY

"It is not the events in our lives that upset us, but rather how we interpret them." — **Epictetus**

Emotions are powerful. They can push you forward or hold you back. In fitness, they show up in every corner of the journey: frustration when progress feels slow, disappointment after a missed goal, complacency when motivation fades. These feelings are natural, but if left unchecked, they can derail you.

The Stoics teach us that while we can't control what happens to us, we can control how we respond. Mastering your emotions isn't about suppressing them—it's about understanding them, managing them, and using them to fuel your growth.

Why Emotional Mastery Matters In Fitness

Every fitness journey has its highs and lows. Some days, you feel unstoppable. Other days, you struggle just to show up. Emotional mastery is what keeps you consistent through it all.

It's not about ignoring your feelings—it's about not letting them dictate your actions. Whether you're frustrated by a bad workout or discouraged by a lack of progress, emotional mastery helps you stay grounded and focused. It allows you to keep moving forward, no matter how you feel in the moment.

How To Master Your Emotions

1. Practice Mindfulness

When frustration or discouragement arises, take a moment to pause. Breathe deeply and acknowledge your feelings without judgment. This simple act of mindfulness creates space between the emotion and your reaction, helping you respond with clarity instead of impulse.

2. Focus on What You Can Control

A bad workout, a missed goal, a tough day—these things happen. Instead of dwelling on what you can't change, ask yourself: *"What can I do right now?"* Focus on your effort, your attitude, and your next step. When you narrow your focus to what's within your control, emotions lose their grip.

3. Channel Emotions into Action

Feeling frustrated? Use that energy to push harder in your workout. Feeling anxious? Go for a run to clear your mind. By channeling your emotions into productive action, you take control of how they affect you. Emotions aren't your enemy— they're your fuel.

A Real-Life Example: Turning Bad Emotions Into Growth

There was a time when anxiety was taking over. I was so caught up worrying about the future that I couldn't focus on what actually mattered that day. It was frustrating. I felt stuck, like everything I had to do was harder than it really was.

Then I came across something Marcus Aurelius wrote: "Confine yourself to the present." That made sense. I couldn't change the future, but I could decide what to do today.

So, I started focusing on what I could control: getting to the gym, eating better, and working on my mindset. It wasn't a quick fix, but the more I stuck to it, the better I felt. Taking care of those small, daily actions made me feel stronger—physically and mentally.

Reflection: How Do Emotions Shape Your Journey?

Take a moment to think about your own fitness journey:

- *Have frustration or disappointment ever led you to give up or skip a workout?*
- *How can you respond differently the next time those emotions arise?*
- *What emotions can you channel into action today?*

Mastering your emotions isn't about eliminating them—it's about harnessing them. It's about recognizing that you have the power to choose your response, no matter what you feel.

"Emotions don't have to control you. Use them, direct them, and let them push you toward your goals." — **Matheus Lourenco**

From Emotional Mastery to Strength in Adversity

Mastering your emotions empowers you to remain calm and composed, but adversity is where true strength is forged. Let's explore how challenges and setbacks can become the building blocks of resilience.

CHAPTER 10: STRENGTH IN ADVERSITY

Adversity is a certainty. Whether it's a fitness journey or life itself, challenges will come. An injury might force you to slow down. A plateau might test your patience. Some days, it will feel like the universe is working against you.

The Stoics would tell you: good. Adversity isn't something to fear —it's something to use. It's the fire that forges resilience, the weight that builds your inner strength. The way you face these moments defines your progress, not just in the gym, but in life.

Why Adversity Is Essential

Think about a time when everything seemed easy. Did it really push you to grow? Probably not. Growth comes from the struggle —from facing something hard and coming out stronger on the other side.

In fitness, setbacks like injuries or missed goals feel discouraging. But they're also opportunities. A plateau might teach you to refine your technique. An injury might force you to strengthen overlooked areas. These challenges, when embraced, shape you into someone more disciplined, resilient, and determined.

How To Build Strength Through Adversity

1. Reframe Setbacks as Opportunities

When adversity strikes, stop and ask yourself: *What can I learn from this? How can this make me stronger?*

A bad workout isn't a failure—it's feedback. An injury isn't the end—it's a chance to focus on something new. When you reframe setbacks, they stop being roadblocks and become stepping stones.

2. Responding to Adversity

Adversity isn't here to derail you—it's here to test you. When setbacks disrupt your progress, the challenge isn't to do what you planned, but to do what you can. If an injury forces you to slow down, use the time to reflect, refine your strategy, or strengthen overlooked areas. Each obstacle is a teacher, pushing you to grow in ways you might not have chosen—but that you need.

Resilience is born not from avoiding hardship but from facing it head-on. When adversity strikes, it's not a signal to stop—it's a call to rise, adapt, and keep moving forward in whatever way you can.

3. Stay Committed to the Process

Adversity tempts you to give up. It whispers, *"What's the point?"*

But strength lies in staying committed, even when it's hard. Remind yourself why you started. Show up, even when it's tough. True progress comes from persistence.

A Real-Life Example: Turning Setbacks Into Strength

A few years ago, when i was at the gym, I let my ego get the best of me. I loaded up more weight on the bench press than I should have, thinking I could handle it. Partway through the lift, I felt a sharp pain in my shoulder. In that moment, I knew I had messed up. My favorite exercise was now off-limits, and I felt defeated.

At first, I was frustrated. Benching was my go-to, and without it, I didn't feel like myself. But instead of quitting, I made a choice: if I couldn't train my upper body, I'd focus on what I'd been neglecting —my legs. Squats, lunges, and other lower-body exercises became my priority.

It wasn't glamorous, and I struggled at first, but as the weeks passed, I started to see progress. My legs, once my weakest area, were getting stronger. When my shoulder finally healed, I came back to the bench press more balanced and determined.

That injury, as frustrating as it was, turned out to be one of the best things that could've happened to me. It forced me to grow in ways I hadn't planned. Sometimes, the things that knock us down are exactly what we need to stand taller.

Reflection: Your Strength In Adversity

Think back to a challenge you've faced in your fitness journey:

- *How did you respond?*
- *What lessons did you take from the experience?*

> • *How can you approach adversity differently in the future?*

Adversity isn't here to defeat you. It's here to teach you. Each setback is a chance to grow stronger, more resilient, and more determined.

"Adversity doesn't block your path—it sharpens it. Use it, and you'll discover strength you never knew you had." **— Matheus Lourenco**

From Strength in Adversity to Perspective in Fitness

Adversity challenges you to grow stronger, but how you perceive those challenges shapes your journey. In the next chapter, we'll explore the role of perspective in transforming setbacks into opportunities for growth.

CHAPTER 11: PERSPECTIVE SHAPES PROGRESS

"The happiness of your life depends upon the quality of your thoughts." — **Marcus Aurelius**

Perspective shapes everything. It's the lens through which you see the world, and in fitness, it can mean the difference between giving up and pushing forward. A setback can feel like failure—or it can be a chance to grow. Progress can feel slow—or it can remind you of how far you've come.

The Stoics understood that perspective isn't just about what happens to you; it's about how you choose to interpret it. And in fitness, that choice can transform the way you approach every workout, every goal, and every challenge.

Why Perspective Matters

Imagine two people facing the same obstacle: a plateau in their fitness progress. One feels defeated, questioning why they even bother. The other sees it as a chance to reassess, refine, and improve.

What's the difference? Perspective.

Stoicism teaches us to see every experience as an opportunity to practice resilience, patience, and self-mastery. When you shift your perspective, setbacks stop being roadblocks and become steppingstones.

How To Cultivate A Positive Perspective

1. Practice Gratitude

When progress feels slow or challenges feel overwhelming, pause and ask: *What am I grateful for today?* Maybe it's the strength you've already built, the energy you feel, or even just the fact that you showed up. Gratitude shifts your focus from what's missing to what's present, helping you see your journey as a gift rather than a burden.

2. Reframe Negative Thoughts

Negative thoughts will come—that's human. But you don't have to believe them. When you hear, *"I'm not strong enough,"* challenge it. Say instead, *"I'm getting stronger every day."* This isn't about blind optimism—it's about choosing a perspective that empowers rather than limits you.

3. Focus on the Bigger Picture

Why did you start this journey? What are you working toward? Reminding yourself of your "why" keeps you grounded when the day-to-day feels hard. Maybe today's workout wasn't perfect, but it's one step closer to your long-term goal. Perspective helps you see the forest, not just the trees.

Real-Life Example: Shifting To Gratitude

I used to get frustrated about not having enough time to train. "What's the point?" I'd think. "30 minutes won't change anything." It annoyed me so much that I'd skip workouts altogether.

But one day, I caught myself. I thought, "At least I have 30 minutes. That's enough to do something." So, I went to the gym. I didn't waste time. I warmed up, pushed myself through a short but intense session, and left feeling accomplished.

That was the shift. I stopped seeing 30 minutes as "not enough" and started treating it as a chance to move forward. It taught me that it's not about having the perfect conditions—it's about making the most of what you have.

Reflection: Your Perspective Shapes Your Journey

Take a moment to think about your own fitness journey:

- *Are there moments where a negative perspective has held you back?*
- *What thoughts could you reframe to create a more positive mindset?*
- *How can gratitude or your "why" help you see challenges differently?*

Perspective isn't about ignoring difficulties—it's about choosing how you see them. When you shift your perspective, you gain the power to turn every challenge into an opportunity, every step into progress, and every moment into a chance to grow.

"Your thoughts shape your reality. Shift your perspective, and you'll transform your journey." — **Matheus Lourenco**

From Perspective to Recovery

The way you view challenges shapes your journey, but growth also requires knowing when to pause. As we explore the next chapter, we'll discover how rest isn't a break from progress—it's the foundation for achieving your goals.

CHAPTER 12: THE POWER OF RECOVERY

"If one oversteps the bounds of moderation, the greatest pleasures cease to please." — **Epictetus**

In the world of fitness, rest is often misunderstood. We celebrate effort, consistency, and discipline—but rest? That feels like weakness. Yet, the truth is, rest isn't just a pause in your progress —it's where the real progress happens.

The Stoics believed in balance. They taught that overindulgence, even in something positive, leads to diminishing returns. The same is true in fitness. Without proper recovery, your body can't rebuild, and your mind can't recharge. Rest isn't the opposite of hard work—it's part of it.

Why Rest Matters

Think about your hardest workout. Every rep, every sprint, every ounce of effort creates micro-tears in your muscles. That's the stress your body needs to grow. But the growth doesn't happen during the workout—it happens after.

When you rest, your body repairs itself. It strengthens muscles, restores energy, and prepares you for the next challenge. Ignore rest, and you risk overtraining, burnout, and even injury. Embrace it, and you'll discover that rest is the secret weapon of sustainable progress.

How To Embrace Rest And Recovery

1. Plan Rest Days

Don't leave rest to chance—schedule it. At least one or two days each week should be dedicated to recovery. These aren't wasted days. Light activities like walking or yoga can keep you active without straining your body.

2. Prioritize Sleep

Sleep isn't optional—it's essential. During sleep, your body releases growth hormones, repairs muscles, and recharges your mind. Aim for 7-9 hours of quality sleep each night. Sleep isn't a luxury; it's your most powerful recovery tool.

3. Listen to Your Body

Your body knows when it's had enough—are you listening? Persistent fatigue, irritability, or declining performance are red flags. Rest isn't a sign of weakness; it's a sign of wisdom. Pay attention, and give your body the care it needs.

Real-Life Example: Rest As A Tool For Growth

There was a time when I was working a tough, physical job and trying to train every single day. I thought that was what it meant to be dedicated—show up no matter what. But after a while, I started to notice something. I was exhausted. My workouts felt heavy, my progress stalled, and I just wasn't performing the way I wanted to.

Eventually, I realized the problem wasn't my effort—it was my recovery. So, I made a change. I scaled back to three gym sessions a week and let myself rest on the other days. At first, it felt wrong, like I wasn't doing enough. But then, something changed. My energy came back. My strength improved. I started hitting goals I hadn't reached in months.

That experience taught me something simple but powerful: rest isn't taking a step back. It's giving your body the chance to move forward stronger than ever.

Reflection: Rest As Strength

Pause and think:

- *Are you giving yourself enough time to recover?*
- *Do you see rest as part of your progress, or as a weakness?*
- *How can you make rest a more intentional part of your journey?*

Rest isn't the absence of effort—it's what makes effort sustainable. By embracing recovery, you allow your body and mind to recharge, ensuring that you show up stronger, every single day.

"*Rest isn't a break from progress—it's the foundation of it. Embrace recovery, and you'll see just how far it can take you.*" — **Matheus Lourenco**

From Rest to Legacy

Rest allows you to rebuild and grow stronger, but what you do with that strength is what truly matters. In the next chapter, we'll explore how your actions today can shape the legacy you leave behind.

CHAPTER 13: YOUR FITNESS LEGACY

"The best way to predict the future is to create it." — **Peter Drucker**

Fitness isn't just about the body—it's about the example you set, the values you live by, and the impact you leave behind. For the Stoics, living a virtuous life meant acting with purpose and integrity in all things. Your fitness journey is no exception.

Every time you show up, push through, and stay disciplined, you're not just building your own strength—you're inspiring those around you. Your journey is a ripple effect, creating positive change that extends far beyond yourself.

Why Your Fitness Journey Matters

Your actions have more power than you realize. When you stay committed to your goals, it's not just about what you achieve—it's about who you become and how you inspire others.

Imagine a friend who watches you prioritize your health. Over time, they're encouraged to take their first steps toward fitness. Maybe a family member sees your dedication and starts making healthier choices. Your journey has the potential to motivate, uplift, and transform others.

The Stoics believed in leading by example. In fitness, that means showing others what's possible when you combine discipline, perseverance, and self-care.

How To Leave A Positive Fitness Legacy

1. Lead by Example

Words are powerful, but actions speak louder. Let your dedication to fitness demonstrate the value of consistency and hard work. Whether it's showing up for workouts, eating mindfully, or setting ambitious goals, your behavior inspires more than any advice you could give.

2. Share Your Story

Every fitness journey is unique, filled with struggles, breakthroughs, and lessons. By sharing your story—whether online, in conversations, or even casually—you can show others that progress is possible. Your vulnerability and honesty might be the spark someone else needs to start their own journey.

3. Encourage and Support Others

Fitness isn't a solo endeavor. Celebrate the wins of those around you. Offer encouragement when they face challenges. By being a source of positivity and support, you create an environment where others can thrive.

A Real-Life Example: The Ripple Effect Of Commitment

When I first started going to the gym, no one really cared. Honestly, some people even made fun of me. "Why bother?" "You'll quit in a few weeks." I tried to brush it off, but those words stuck with me. Still, I kept going. Day after day, I showed up, even when no one believed in what I was doing.

At first, nothing changed. Progress was slow, and I wasn't sure if it was even worth it. But then, little by little, things started to shift. My body changed. My energy improved. People around me started noticing. The same ones who doubted me were now asking, "What are you doing?" "How can I start?"

That's when it hit me: my consistency wasn't just changing me—it was inspiring others. What started as a personal journey became something bigger. I never set out to motivate anyone, but by sticking to my goals, I showed people what was possible.

Reflection: What Legacy Will You Leave?

Pause for a moment and think:

- *How has your fitness journey influenced those around you?*
- *What example do you want to set for others?*
- *How can you use your story to inspire positive change?*

Your fitness journey isn't just about you. It's about the inspiration you provide, the lessons you share, and the impact you create. Every workout, every decision, and every step forward is a chance to leave a legacy that lasts far beyond your own life.

"The strongest thing you'll ever build isn't your body—it's the example you set. Live your journey with purpose, and you'll inspire others to do the same." — **Matheus Lourenco**

From Legacy to Mindfulness

Your legacy isn't just what you leave behind—it's the impact you make every day. To make that impact meaningful, you need to be present in each moment. In the next chapter, we'll explore how Stoic mindfulness can help you stay grounded and intentional in your fitness journey and beyond.

CHAPTER 14: MINDFULNESS IN MOTION

"Nowhere can man find a quieter or more untroubled retreat than in his own soul." — **Marcus Aurelius**

In a world filled with distractions, it's easy to lose sight of the moment. Fitness, like life, demands presence. Yet, how often do we find ourselves rushing through reps, checking our phones, or letting our minds wander during a workout? Stoic mindfulness offers an antidote—a way to anchor ourselves to the present and engage fully with what we're doing, right here and right now.

For the Stoics, mindfulness wasn't a trendy practice; it was a necessity. To be mindful is to live deliberately, free from regrets about the past or anxieties about the future. In fitness, this means focusing not on the result, but on the process—each breath, each movement, each step forward.

Why Mindfulness Matters In Fitness

Mindfulness isn't just for meditation—it's a powerful tool for enhancing performance, preventing injuries, and building mental clarity. When you approach your workout with full presence, you unlock its true potential.

1. Improve Performance

When you focus entirely on each rep, you're not just going through the motions—you're engaging your body and mind fully, maximizing the impact of every movement.

2. Prevent Injuries

A wandering mind leads to mistakes. By staying present, you ensure proper form and technique, reducing the risk of injury.

3. Sharpen Mental Clarity

Fitness isn't just physical—it's mental. Quieting distractions allows you to make deliberate, purposeful choices, whether it's pacing yourself during a run or pushing harder during a lift.

How To Practice Mindfulness In Fitness

1. Focus on Your Breathing

Your breath is a powerful anchor. Before a lift, inhale deeply to prepare your body. Exhale as you push through. This simple practice keeps you grounded and improves your performance.

2. Eliminate Distractions

Put your phone away. Listen to the sounds around you—the weights clinking, your breath, your footsteps. Feel the sensation of your muscles working. Presence is found in these details.

3. Set Intentions Before Your Workout

Begin each session with a question: *What do I want to achieve today?* This intention aligns your effort with purpose, keeping you focused throughout.

Mindfulness Through Reflection

Mindfulness doesn't end when the workout is over. By reflecting on your session, you can identify areas of growth and celebrate small victories.

- *Did I improve my form?*
- *Did I lift heavier? Run farther?*
- *What felt challenging, and what can I adjust next time?*

Reflection turns your workout into a learning experience, building both your body and your mind.

The Stoic Perspective On Mindfulness

Marcus Aurelius reminds us: "Confine yourself to the present." For the Stoics, the present moment was all that truly mattered.
In fitness, this means letting go of distractions—don't dwell on yesterday's missed workout or worry about tomorrow's goals. Focus on the task at hand. The effort you make today is what shapes the results you'll see in the future.

Reflection: Bringing Mindfulness Into Your Fitness

Take a moment to ask yourself:

- *How often do I let distractions pull me away from the present during a workout?*

- *What can I do to focus more fully on the now?*
- *How can I use mindfulness to improve both my performance and my experience?*

Mindfulness isn't about perfection—it's about presence. By bringing your full attention to each moment, you turn your fitness journey into something more than physical progress—it becomes a practice in living deliberately, with purpose and intention.

"In the quiet focus of the present, you unlock the true potential of your body and mind." — Matheus Lourenco

From Mindfulness to Temperance

Mindfulness keeps you grounded in the present, but true balance requires more than awareness—it calls for moderation. In the next chapter, we'll explore how temperance guides your choices, helping you find harmony in both fitness and life

CHAPTER 15: THE BALANCE OF MODERATION

"The virtue of temperance is not in saying 'no' to everything but in knowing when to say 'yes.'" — **Marcus Aurelius**

Why Moderation Matters:

Let's be honest—alcohol can feel like a reward, a way to relax, or even just a way to fit in socially. But if we're not careful, it can creep into our routine and start taking more than it gives. Whether it's slowing down your progress in fitness or leaving you feeling less sharp mentally, overindulging never leads to anything great.

The truth is, moderation isn't about being perfect; it's about being intentional. If you want to build a strong body and a clear mind, you can't let anything, including alcohol, take over.

The Stoic Perspective:

The Stoics were big on balance. They weren't about cutting out every pleasure but about making sure those pleasures didn't control them. Marcus Aurelius said it best: "You have power over your mind—not outside events." That applies to a lot, but it definitely works with alcohol. You don't have to quit entirely to stay in control—you just need to make sure you're the one calling the shots.

Moderation isn't weakness; it's strength. It's about enjoying life without letting those moments of enjoyment derail your bigger goals.

Real-Life Example: Temperance In Action: My Story

For a long time, I didn't really think about alcohol—I just drank. It was my way of unwinding, of escaping stress. From my twenties into my early thirties, it became a pattern. But when I started focusing on my fitness and embracing stoicism, I realized I couldn't keep going like that.

I didn't quit drinking altogether, but I changed my relationship with it. Now, when I have a drink, it's intentional. I've learned that you don't have to give something up entirely to feel in control—you just have to shift how you think about it. And trust me, the clarity and progress I gained were worth it.

Practical Actions For Moderation:

Get Honest About Your Habits:
Ask yourself: Why do I drink? Is it stress? Social pressure? Boredom? Once you know your "why," it's easier to take control.

Set Some Rules (and Stick to Them):
Maybe it's saving drinks for special occasions or limiting yourself to one or two. Whatever works for you, stick to it.

Find Better Outlets:
If you're drinking to relax or escape, replace it with something healthier. A workout, a good book, or even a walk can do wonders.

Final Reflection

Here's the thing: true freedom isn't about cutting out every little indulgence—it's about making sure they don't control you. Moderation isn't deprivation; it's knowing what really matters and aligning your actions with those priorities.

"Balance in life includes enjoying a drink, but never letting it cloud your purpose." — **Matheus Lourenco**

Balance Is the Antidote to Comparison
We've talked about balancing what's inside your glass. Now, let's talk about balancing what's inside your mind. Comparisons can be tricky—they can motivate us or drain us. In the next chapter, we'll dive into how to handle them in a way that helps you move forward without losing your focus.

CHAPTER 16: BEYOND COMPARISON

"If you want to improve, be content to be thought foolish and stupid."
— **Epictetus**

It starts small—watching someone at the gym lifting more than you thought possible, scrolling past a perfect transformation photo online, or hearing about a friend smashing personal records. At first, it's just a spark of curiosity, but soon it grows. You start to wonder: *Why am I not there yet? Why does it look so easy for them?*

Comparison has a way of stealing your focus and turning progress into frustration. You stop celebrating your wins because they don't feel big enough. You forget the strides you've made because someone else's journey seems better.

But Stoicism reminds us to resist this trap. Epictetus knew that growth isn't found in others' achievements. It's found in your own discipline, your own effort. Your only competition is the person you were yesterday.

Why Comparison Holds You Back

Comparison feels natural, but it rarely helps. What you're seeing —their PR, their perfect physique, their confident smile—isn't the full picture. You don't see the struggles they've faced or the setbacks they've overcome. You don't know the doubts they've battled in private.

And while you're focused on someone else's story, you're missing out on your own. You're giving energy to something outside of your control instead of focusing on what truly matters: the effort you bring to your journey.

The Stoics teach us that the only measure worth using is the one you create for yourself. What others achieve is irrelevant to your growth. What you achieve? That's everything.

How To Let Go Of Comparison

1. Turn Your Focus Inward

Stop looking at what others are doing and start looking at what you've accomplished. Ask yourself:

- *What progress have I made this week?*
- *Am I stronger, faster, or more consistent than I was a month ago?*

Every step forward—no matter how small—is a victory.

2. Curate Your Environment

Social media often fuels comparison. If scrolling makes you feel inadequate, change the narrative. Follow accounts that inspire you, not ones that create unrealistic pressure. Surround yourself with people who celebrate effort, not just results.

3. Practice Daily Gratitude

Instead of fixating on what you haven't achieved, celebrate what your body can do today. Maybe you ran your first mile, hit a new PR, or just showed up when it was hard. Gratitude shifts your perspective, grounding you in the present and reminding you how far you've already come.

Real-Life Example: Perspective

I remember meeting a guy at the gym—I'll call him Jake. Jake was one of those people who seemed to have it all together. His lifts were impressive, his confidence unshakable. Meanwhile, I was struggling with basics.

One day, I worked up the courage to talk to him. I told him how much I admired his progress. Jake laughed, shook his head, and said, "You didn't see me three years ago when I could barely squat an empty bar. This? This took time. Keep going. You're already ahead of where I started."

That stuck with me. What looked effortless wasn't. What felt unattainable was just a few steps further down the same road I was on.

Reflection: Your Journey, Your Rules

Take a moment to reflect:

- *Where has comparison held you back?*
- *What progress have you made that deserves celebration?*
- *How can you shift your focus inward, starting today?*

Comparison doesn't make you stronger—it makes you doubt the

strength you already have. When you let it go, you reclaim the energy to focus on your own growth. You see your wins for what they are: proof that you're moving forward.

"Your only competition is the person you were yesterday—focus there, and you'll always progress." — **Matheus Lourenco**

From Comparison to embracing the journey

Growth doesn't come from chasing someone else's path. It comes from walking your own. The process isn't always glamorous, and it often feels slow, but it is in the process itself that true victory is found. Let's explore how embracing the journey leads to lasting success

CHAPTER 17: VICTORY IN THE PROCESS

"The end is never worth so much as the means." — **Zeno of Citium**

It's easy to fixate on the finish line. You set a goal—whether it's losing weight, running a marathon, or hitting a personal best—and everything becomes about reaching that milestone. But what happens when you get there? The finish line is fleeting. The medal goes in a drawer. The number on the scale becomes just that—a number.

The Stoics teach us something profound: the real victory isn't found in the end result. It's found in the process. Every step you take, every ounce of effort you put in, every moment you choose to show up—those are the true triumphs.

The Stoic Mindset: Process Over Outcome

1. Focus on Effort, Not Results

The Stoics believed that outcomes are outside of our control, but effort is always within it. You can't force the scale to drop a certain number, but you can control what you eat today. You can't guarantee a PR, but you can show up and give your best in training. When you focus on the process, you free yourself from the pressure of perfection.

2. Embrace the Process as a Victory

Victory isn't a trophy you hold at the end of the journey—it's the effort you put in along the way. Each decision to move forward, every challenge you face with determination, and every moment you honor your commitment is success in itself.

Instead of waiting for some distant finish line, see the process as its own reward. The daily grind shapes you. The struggle refines you. True triumph lies in showing up and pushing yourself, even when no one is watching.

How To Embrace The Process

1. Track Effort, Not Just Results

Keep a journal, but don't just record the weight you lifted or the miles you ran. Write down the effort you put in—the days you showed up when you didn't feel like it, the small improvements in form or endurance. Over time, these efforts add up to something far greater than numbers.

2. Practice Gratitude Along the Way

At the end of each day, reflect on how your actions aligned with your values. Did you show discipline? Did you make progress, no matter how small? Gratitude keeps you grounded, reminding you that the process itself is a privilege.

3. Redefine Success

Success isn't about reaching a single goal—it's about continuing the journey, even when it gets tough. True success is found in persistence, not perfection.

Real-Life Example: Finding Joy In The Process

When I started working out, it wasn't anything impressive. I wasn't lifting heavy weights or running long distances. I'd go to the gym, spend 20 minutes on the treadmill, and maybe do a few sets of weights. It felt small, but it was a start.

At first, it didn't seem like much was changing. I didn't notice big improvements, and I'd see other people making faster progress. But I kept showing up. Little by little, I started to feel stronger. My energy improved, and I realized I actually enjoyed the routine.

I never entered a competition or chased dramatic results, but that didn't matter. The small steps I took every day were enough. For me, the process became the reward.

Reflection: Redefining Your Own Victory

Take a moment to reflect:

- *Do you measure success only by the end result?*
- *What small wins can you celebrate today?*
- *How can you shift your focus to embrace the process itself?*

The Stoics remind us that the journey is where life happens. The daily commitment, the moments of effort, the choices to keep going even when it's hard—that's where true strength is built.

"The finish line is just a moment. The process is the legacy you carry with you every day." — **Matheus Lourenco**

From Process to Mental Fortitude

The process builds patience, but true growth comes when we strengthen our minds to face any challenge. Let's dive into how cultivating mental fortitude can help us overcome obstacles and thrive under pressure.

CHAPTER 18: BUILDING MENTAL FORTITUDE

You are a little soul carrying around a corpse." — **Marcus Aurelius**

1. Treat Physical Challenges as Mental Training

The next time you're tempted to stop mid-workout, pause. Remind yourself that this is an opportunity to practice resilience. Push through one more set, one more rep, one more step. Each effort makes your mind stronger, more resilient.

2. Set Challenges That Scare You

Growth doesn't come from comfort. Create fitness goals that feel intimidating—whether it's trying a new class, lifting heavier weights, or running farther than you ever have. Facing these challenges head-on strengthens your resolve, making you braver in the gym and in life.

3. Stay Grounded in the Present

When the workout gets tough, it's easy to let your mind wander to how much more you have to do. Instead, focus on the now.

Pay attention to your breathing, your form, and the movement of your body. Staying present keeps you in control, even when things feel overwhelming.

A Real-Life Example: Turning Obstacles Into Opportunities

I used to think I needed everything to be perfect in order to succeed—perfect conditions, perfect timing. But the more I waited for the "perfect moment," the more I put things off.

Then, I realized something: obstacles weren't a reason to quit; they were opportunities to adapt. One day, when I couldn't hit the gym due to a busy schedule, I used that time to take a walk outside. I realized that the simple act of moving—whether in the gym or outside—kept my vibes going.

That shift in perspective taught me something important: it's not about waiting for perfect conditions, it's about making the most of what you have, right where you are.

Reflection: Strengthening Your Mind Through Your Body

Take a moment to reflect:

- *How has physical fitness helped you grow mentally?*
- *What challenges have you faced that forced you to dig deep and keep going?*
- *How can you use your workouts to build resilience, not just strength?*

The Stoics teach us that the mind is our most powerful tool. The gym is where you sharpen it. Each time you choose to push through discomfort, you prove to yourself that you're stronger than the doubts in your head.

"Physical fitness is the gateway to mental fortitude. Every challenge you overcome in the gym builds the strength to overcome life's obstacles, too." — **Matheus Lourenco**

From Mental Fortitude to Discipline in Nutrition

Mental fortitude empowers your decisions, and nutrition is where discipline truly takes form. Let's explore how your choices at the table reflect your strength and commitment.

CHAPTER 19:
DISCIPLINE IN
NUTRITION

"We must indulge the body only as far as is needed for health." — **Seneca**

Food is everywhere. It's tied to our culture, our celebrations, even our emotions. Yet, every meal you eat is also a choice—a moment where self-discipline either strengthens or weakens. Do you eat to nourish your body and align with your goals? Or do you act on impulse, letting cravings take control?

The Stoics saw every decision as an opportunity to live by their principles. Eating is no different. It's not just an act of survival—it's a practice in discipline, moderation, and gratitude. When you approach nutrition with intention, you're not just feeding your body—you're shaping your character.

The Stoic Principles Of Eating

1. Act on Reason, Not Cravings

Impulse tells you to grab the candy bar or eat mindlessly while scrolling through your phone. Reason steps in and asks: *Does this choice serve my goals?* A Stoic doesn't reject enjoyment, but they make decisions with intention. They choose food that sustains their health and aligns with their purpose.

2. Indulge with Moderation

Indulgence isn't failure—it's part of being human. But indulgence without restraint becomes a habit, and habits shape who we are. A Stoic treats indulgence as a conscious choice, savoring it without guilt and returning to discipline the next moment.

How To Bring Stoic Discipline To Nutrition

1. Simplify Your Choices

You don't need the perfect diet plan to eat well. Instead, focus on simplicity. Choose whole, minimally processed foods that energize you and align with your values. Complexity isn't the answer—consistency is.

2. Create a Supportive Environment

Willpower isn't infinite. Don't leave yourself at the mercy of temptation. Stock your kitchen with foods that fuel your body and limit the presence of things that derail you. By shaping your environment, you make discipline easier to maintain.

3. Practice Gratitude Before Meals

Before eating, pause. Reflect on the journey of your food—the farmers who grew it, the resources that transported it, the effort that prepared it. Gratitude grounds you in the moment, making every meal a reminder of how much you have to be thankful for.

Real-Life Example: Changing Habits Changed My Life

For years, I tried every diet you can think of. Low carb, high protein, juice cleanses—none of them lasted. I'd lose a few pounds, but I always ended up feeling worse and more drained.

Then, I stopped. I stopped chasing quick fixes and focused on something simple: real food. Vegetables, lean meat, healthy fats. It wasn't glamorous, but it worked.

I started feeling better almost immediately. More energy, better workouts, and my body started changing. It wasn't about being perfect—it was about making better choices every day. Real food gave me the energy to keep going, and it changed my body in ways those crazy diets never did.

Reflection: Food As A Practice Of Discipline

Take a moment to reflect:

- *Are your eating habits aligned with your goals?*
- *Do you eat mindfully, or do emotions drive your choices?*
- *How can you bring more intention and gratitude to your meals?*

Food isn't just about nourishment—it's about choice. Every meal is a chance to practice discipline, to honor your body, and to strengthen your commitment to yourself.

"Discipline isn't found in perfection—it's built in the small, daily choices that align with who you want to become." — **Matheus Lourenco**

These examples and habit changes show that the path to transformation isn't about quick fixes or trendy diets. It's about consistency and conscious choices every day. And in the end, that's what truly makes the difference.

Now, as you reflect on the lessons I've shared, think about how you can apply these principles in your own life. Real growth happens when we stop waiting for the perfect moment and start taking action with what we have, where we are.

CONCLUSION: EMBRACING STOIC STRENGTH IN ALL ASPECTS OF LIFE

"Waste no more time arguing about what a good man should be. Be one." — **Marcus Aurelius**

As we finish this journey together, take a moment to think about how far you've come. This book wasn't just about building physical strength or improving fitness—it was about becoming someone who faces challenges head-on, who chooses resilience over resignation, and who knows their own power to shape their life.

The lessons of Stoicism—wisdom, courage, justice, and temperance—aren't abstract ideas. They're habits. They show up every time you choose effort over excuses, discipline over distractions, and courage over fear. Fitness is just one part of the story. What you've built here—the mindset, the focus, the patience—will guide you in so many other areas of life.

Carrying Stoic Strength Into Life

When you think about the challenges ahead—whether in your work, relationships, or personal growth—remember the strength you've already shown. You didn't just strengthen your body on this journey; you fortified your mind and heart, too.

Every workout, every healthy choice, every moment when you kept going even when it felt hard—that's where your strength came from. It's not in perfection or quick results. It's in the process, the showing up, the doing. That's what will continue to carry you forward.

A Personal Word Of Gratitude

Writing this book has been one of the most meaningful things I've ever done because it's about sharing the lessons that helped me when I needed them most. To know that these pages have been a part of your journey—it's a gift I don't take lightly.

If this book inspired or helped you in any way, I'd love it if you shared your thoughts in a review. Your voice matters, and your feedback could help someone else discover this book and take the first step in their own transformation.

Thank you for letting me be part of your story.

A Final Reflection

"A room without books is like a body without a soul." — ***Cicero***

Let this book be more than something you read once. Let it become part of how you live. True strength isn't found in a number on a scale or a trophy on a shelf—it's in every small choice to move forward, to keep growing, and to honor your values.

When life gets heavy, remember what you've already overcome. When you stumble, get back up. When you face a challenge, lean into it. That's what it means to live with Stoic strength: to embrace life as it is, and to use every experience to grow.

Carry these lessons with you, not just in the gym but everywhere. Approach your days with courage, kindness, and gratitude. And remember, it's not about reaching the end—it's about who you become along the way.

"True strength isn't in what you achieve. It's in the person you're becoming. And you, my friend, are just getting started."

ABOUT THE AUTHOR

Six years ago, I stepped off a plane in Australia with nothing but a backpack, some big dreams, and absolutely no English. It was just me and the overwhelming idea that I had to rebuild my life from scratch. It wasn't easy. In fact, it was terrifying. Being alone in a foreign place, unable to ask for something as simple as a glass of water, was one of the hardest challenges I'd ever faced. But over time, I learned that discomfort is one of life's greatest teachers.

I stumbled upon stoicism during that journey, almost by accident. It felt like the ancient philosophers were speaking directly to me: "Focus on what you can control. Accept the rest. And above all, keep moving forward." These words helped me overcome the language barrier, the loneliness, and the constant fear of failure. More than that, they taught me to see every obstacle as a steppingstone.

At the same time, I found fitness as a way to put these lessons into action. Lifting weights, running, and training became more than just physical activities; they were mental challenges. Every rep was a test of discipline. Every run was a reminder that growth comes from pushing through discomfort.

This book is the result of that journey—a blend of stoic philosophy and practical lessons learned in the gym and in life. My hope is that it helps you overcome your own challenges, build resilience, and find strength you didn't know you had.

And if there's one thing I've learned, it's this: no matter where you start, no matter how hard it feels, progress is always possible. You just have to take the first step.